BEI GRIN MACHT SICH IHR WISSEN BEZAHLT

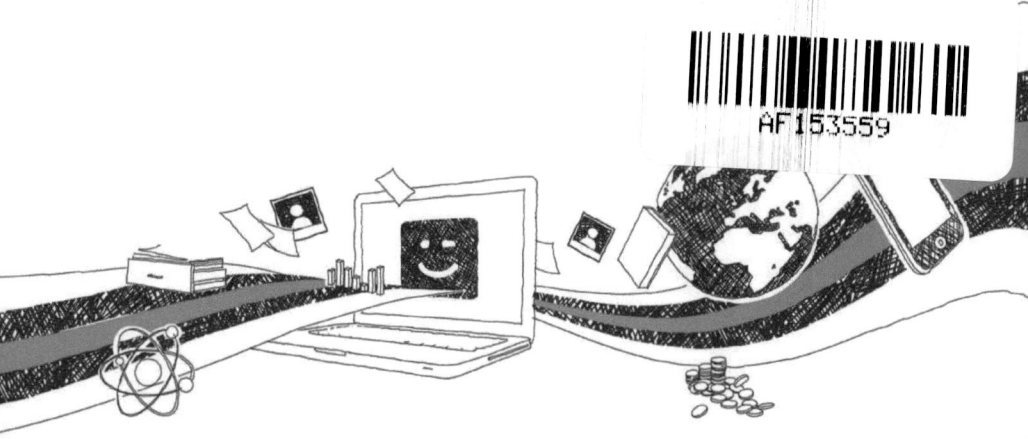

- Wir veröffentlichen Ihre Hausarbeit, Bachelor- und Masterarbeit

- Ihr eigenes eBook und Buch - weltweit in allen wichtigen Shops

- Verdienen Sie an jedem Verkauf

Jetzt bei www.GRIN.com hochladen und kostenlos publizieren

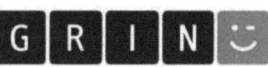

Can machine learning models be used to categorize breast cancer stages reliably?

Marlene Depper

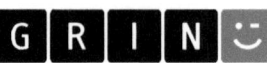

Bibliografische Information der Deutschen Nationalbibliothek:

Die Deutsche Nationalbibliothek verzeichnet diese Publikation in der Deutschen Nationalbibliografie; detaillierte bibliografische Daten sind im Internet über http://dnb.d-nb.de abrufbar.

ISBN: 9783346690326
Dieses Buch ist auch als E-Book erhältlich.

Druck und Bindung: Books on Demand GmbH, Norderstedt Germany
Gedruckt auf säurefreiem Papier aus verantwortungsvollen Quellen

Das vorliegende Werk wurde sorgfältig erarbeitet. Dennoch übernehmen Autoren und Verlag für die Richtigkeit von Angaben, Hinweisen, Links und Ratschlägen sowie eventuelle Druckfehler keine Haftung.

Das Buch bei GRIN: https://www.grin.com/document/1254158

Hochschule für Oekonomie & Management (FOM)
Hochschulzentrum Bonn

Terms Paper

Big Data & Data Science

Topic: Classification of breast cancer stages based on a
                       Convolutional Neural Network

Submitted by: Marlene Elisabeth Depper

submitted on: 27.02.2022

Contents

List of Figures

The figures 1-5 have been removed by GRIN for copyright reasons.

Listings

List of Abbreviations

API   Applitation Programming Interface

CUDA   Compute Unified Device Architecture

CNN   Convolutional Neural Networks

CPU   Central Processing Unit

CRISP-DM   Cross-industry standard process for data mining

GPU   Graphics Processing Unit

ML   Machine Learning

1 Introduction

In 2021, about 34% of adults considered cancer, along with the current COVID-19 pandemic, as one of the biggest health problems in their country.[1] The 5 most dangerous cancers include lung, colorectum, liver, stomach, and breast.

https://www.statista.com/statistics/917148/leading-health-problems-worldwide/

This figure has been removed by GRIN for copyright reasons.

Figure 1: New cancer cases worldwide[2]

As shown in figure 1, breast cancer was the most frequently diagnosed cancer case worldwide, closely followed by lung cancer. In 2020, approximately 2.261.419 new cases of breast cancer were detected.[3] Worldwide, breast cancer accounted for 6.9% of cancer deaths in that year.[4] Early detection could help reduce this high number of deaths.

1.1 Objective

The use of artificial intelligence in healthcare offers a broad range of new opportunities. Various kinds of analytics are already being widely trialed and can help to reduce fault diagnostics.[5] The purpose of this paper is to develop a possible solution that can assist in the diagnosis of breast cancer. By that, the aim is not to replace doctors

---

[1] cf. Elflein (2021c).
[2] cf. Elflein (2021d).
[3] cf. Elflein (2021a).
[4] cf. Elflein (2021b).
[5] cf. Chase (2020).

altogether. Rather, this solution is intended to provide physicians with a means of assisting in the derivation of appropriate treatment methods. Today, especially in regard to the current Corona pandemic, it is more important than ever to reduce the burden on healthcare workers.

Our work addresses the research question of whether machine learning (Machine Learning (ML)) models can be used to categorize breast cancer stages reliably. For this purpose, the possibility of determining the stages of breast cancer with sufficient accuracy will be investigated.

2 Fundamentals

Due to the fact that the cause of breast cancer keeps being unknown, it is crucial to discover the disease as soon as possible for breast cancer control. Besides, then it can positively rise the treatment, save more lives, and reduce costs.[6] It is very difficult to investigate the success of new breast cancer screening methods and technologies because, on the one hand, this requires a certain number of test subjects who would have to be accompanied for years to actually defend the efficiency of an innovative screening method. Therefore, new screening tests will not be studied on their effect on patient outcome but studied by "establishing characteristics of the tests themselves".[7] "Important test characteristics include sensitivity, specificity, safety, cost, simplicity, and patient and clinician acceptability."[8]

2.1 Breast cancer detection

To introduce the subject, you can see a picture of breast cancer symptoms that can be noticed externally below.

https://greenimaging.net/wp-content/uploads/2018/02/greenimaging-breast-cancer-symptoms-illustration.jpg

This figure has been removed by GRIN for copyright reasons.

Figure 2: Breast Cancer Symptoms[9]

---

[6] cf. Cheng et al. (2010).
[7] cf. Elmore et al. (2005).
[8] Elmore et al. (2005).
[9] Mammogram Green Imaging Affordable MRIs, CT Scan, Mammogramm (n.d)

To diagnose breast cancer as early as possible, efforts are made to investigate the most important risk factors that lead to breast cancer as soon as possible. Taking into account a patient's age is the most important factor in breast cancer. It is well known that increasing age, especially after the age of 50, greatly increases the risk of breast cancer. In addition, mammography, which consists of taking an X-ray photo of the breasts, reduces the mortality rate among breast cancer patients. Also, assuming that therapy options will improve in the future, it is likely that early treatment will have a better prognosis than late treatment.[10]

There are several tests and procedures used to detect breast cancer, such as:

- Breast exam:

- Mammogram:

- Breast ultrasound:

- Removing a sample of breast cells for testing (biopsy):

- Breast magnetic resonance imaging (MRI):

Depending on the patient other tests and procedures can be used. In the following, we will focus on the first three key points mentioned above.[11]

2.1.1 Breast exam

The first way to get symptoms or signs of breast cancer is to have your doctor examine your breasts. The doctor examines both breasts and the lymph nodes in the armpit for lumps or other abnormalities, such as anomalies.[12]

2.1.2 Mammogram

An X-ray of the breast is called a mammogram. For many years breast cancer screening with mammography has been recommended. Most women over 40 years in the United States partake in screening activities.[13] For women with or without symptoms, mammograms may be used as a screening test for breast cancer. Often, a mammogram can detect breast cancer early, even before it appears as a lump. During this time, treatment is likely to be easier.[14] There are two types of mammograms. As mentioned above, the first mammography Method is the Screening mammogram and the second method is the diagnostic mammogram.

---

[10] cf. Jandali and Jiga (2019), s.13.
[11] cf. Staff (2021).
[12] cf. Staff (2021).
[13] cf. Elmore et al. (2005).
[14] cf. medical and team (2022).

- screening mammograms: When women who don't have any symptoms of breast problems undergo a screening mammogram, they check for signs of breast cancer. Breast X-rays are typically taken from two different angles.[15] Mammography compresses each breast horizontally. Two plastic plates are placed between the breasts during a screening mammogram. These plates are then compressed briefly to flatten the breast tissue. Two views usually are taken of each breast. Initially, screening and diagnostic mammograms are the same.

https://greenimaging.net/wp-content/uploads/2018/02/greenimaging-screening-mammograpy-1.jpg

This figure has been removed by GRIN for copyright reasons.

Figure 3: Screening Mammogram[16]

Initially, screening and diagnostic mammograms are the same. "Screening mammograms may be done with 2D or 3D technique. The 3D technique may decrease the need to return for additional imaging since the breast is viewed as 'slices' rather than as overlapping structures. It may also for the same reason allow earlier detection of an abnormality, but there is a tradeoff in increased radiation dose."[17]

- diagnostic mammograms: During a diagnostic examination, the patient is present on site. The examination can be done in 2D or 3D and is performed by a radiologist. If additional views are desired, these will also be obtained from the patient. Diagnostic mammography is used for people who may have symptoms associated with breast cancer, such as nipple discharge or unusual lumps.

---

[15] cf. medical and team (2022).
[16] Mammogram Green Imaging Affordable MRIs, CT Scan, Mammogramm (n.d)
[17] cf. Imaging (2022).

Diagnostic mammograms are more complex than a screening examinations. Several specialized images are shot from different angles. The goal of diagnostic imaging is to confirm abnormalities found during screening mammography or self-examination. Ultrasonography is often performed in conjunction with diagnostic mammography to increase specificity and sensitivity.[18]

2.1.3 Breast ultrasound

"Ultrasound uses sound waves to produce images of structures deep within the body."[19] Ultrasound often used to diagnose a specific problem, may be able to distinguish cysts from solid masses, as well as benign from malignant masses. Despite the fact that ultrasound may detect 3 to 4 additional cases of breast cancer per 1000 women in these increased-risk populations, the use of screening ultrasound in the general population is unknown. As a screening tool, breast ultrasound has limitations because it requires a highly skilled operator. Neither the examination techniques nor interpretation criteria are standardized, and breast ultrasound does not consistently detect microcalcifications. Based on preliminary data, there appears to be a higher rate of false-positive examination results with ultrasound than with mammography alone. For example, the false positive rate (based on solid lesions for ultrasound) ranged from 2.4% to 12.9% and 0.7% to 6% for mammography.[20] In order to detect and classify abnormalities in the breast, ultrasound imaging is one of the most commonly used diagnostic tools. A computer-aided diagnosis (CAD) system is a valuable and effective method of breast cancer detection and classification because it eliminates operator dependency and improves diagnostic accuracy.[21] All in all, it is a winsome supplement to mammography because it is most likely available. Compared to other opportunities of methods, ultrasound is inexpensive and well-tolerated by the patients.[22]

2.2 Image recognition

Image recognition is to be classified in the context of artificial intelligence in Deep Learning and describes the automated, i.e. computer-aided technical ability to classify, analyze and interpret the actually unique ability of objects and scenes with the naked eye. Standardized algorithms for image recognition usually contain characteristics such as optical character recognition, pattern matching or, face recognition.[23] A common and current example is the Face ID function in Apple Inc.'s iOS operating system for unlocking the mobile data terminal. The image processing algorithm recognizes particularly salient things in an image. It filters out the area in which the

---

[18] cf. Imaging (2022).
[19] Staff (2021).
[20] cf. Elmore et al. (2005).
[21] cf. Cheng et al. (2010).
[22] cf. Lee (2009).
[23] cf. Paaß and Hecker (2020), p.119.

---

most known information is in the image and then precisely determines its location. Other, still unknown areas and information are excluded from the machine's analysis for the time being. If other information appears more often in the subsequent images, the algorithm will then also take this into account. In order for the algorithm to be able to take more into account and recognize more, it must be trained to do so through continuous practice, so that it can and will work more perfectly over time. Common challenges for an image recognition algorithm can be presented by a change of perspective in the image. Before, the same thing is shown, but the computer recognizes it as a new situation. The depicted scenery has not changed at all, but only the angle of view. Differences in size in the file format can also have a negative influence on the success rate of the algorithm.[24]

2.3 TensorFlow & Keras

TensorFlow and Keras are both open source softwares which were used in order to realize the project. Therefore the softwares will be shortly introduced.

2.3.1 TensorFlow

TensorFlow was originally developed by a team of researchers and engineers at Google. Initially, it was only intended for internal use, until it was finally released as an open-source license in 2015 and has since been freely accessible to everyone.[25] But what exactly is TensorFlow all about? TensorFlow is a scalable, cross-platform programming interface used to implement and execute machine learning algorithms. It enables the efficient implementation of neural networks and is one of the most widely used deep learning libraries available. By accelerating the training of learning systems, it provides significant improvements in training performance.[26] To improve the training performance of learning models, TensorFlow can be run on both, Central Processing Unit (CPU) (Central Processing Unit) and Graphics Processing Unit (GPU) (Graphics Processing Unit) whilst the biggest performance boost has been seen when using GPUs. So far, only GPUs which are capable of Compute Unified Device Architecture (CUDA) (Compute Unified Device Architecture) are supported. TensorFlow also provides interfaces for many different programming languages, with the Python Applitation Programming Interface (API) currently offering the most complete API.[27] TensorFlow is based on a computation graph consisting of several nodes. Each node represents an operation that uses no or multiple inputs and outputs. Represented by so-called tensors, they execute the inputs and outputs. From a mathematical point of view, tensors are a generalization of scalars, vectors, matrices, etc. For example, a tensor of rank 0 represents a scalar, a tensor of rank 1

---

[24] cf. Paaß and Hecker (2020), p.123.
[25] cf. Raschka and Mirjalili (2021), p. 453.
[26] cf. Raschka and Mirjalili (2021), p.451.
[27] cf. Raschka and Mirjalili (2021), p.453.

represents a vector, a tensor of rank 2 represents a matrix, and a tensor of rank 3 represents a three-dimensional stacked matrix (see Figure 4).[28]

This figure has been removed by GRIN for copyright reasons.

Figure 4: Tensor Rank examples[29]

Values in TensorFlow are stored in NumPy-arrays. By that, tensors can be used to access these arrays. The processing of tensors as well as the organization of the data allows them to be traversed for training purposes. In the first released TensorFlow version, computations were based on the construction of a statically directed graph representing the data flow. In TensorFlow 2.0, on the other hand, the library has been greatly revised, making it much easier to create and train NN models. In addition to static computations, it now supports dynamic computation graphs, which are much more flexible.[30]

2.3.2 Keras

Keras is a high-level API and is used for the development of neural networks. As a user-friendly modular programming interface, it enables the creation of prototypes and the development of complex models with just a few lines of code. Thus, it significantly simplifies the development of NN models. As an integral part of TensorFlow, its modules are accessible via tf. Keras. The previously mentioned

---

[28] cf. Raschka and Mirjalili (2021), p.454.
[29] cf. Raschka and Mirjalili (2021), p.454
[30] cf. Raschka and Mirjalili (2021), p.454.

TensorFlow 2.0 already offers tf. Keras is the primary recommended approach for implementing models, supporting TensorFlow-specific functionalities. The use of tf. Keras.Sequential() allows creating a network by stacking layers. Alternatively, the .add() method can be used for this purpose. Better control over the passing of data is enabled by defining a call() method for the model class. For this purpose, the path is explicitly specified. To compile and train these models, the .compile() and .fit() methods can be used.[31]

---

[31] cf. Raschka and Mirjalili (2021), pp. 478-479.

3 Methodology

A methodology often used to analyze data sets in data mining. In this work, different objects are recognized within a large amount of image data sets, the scenery is analyzed and classified accordingly using approaches from said data mining methodology.[32] For this purpose, the approaches of the Cross-industries standard process in Data Mining (Cross-industry standard process for data mining (CRISP-DM) for short) are used in this work.

3.1 CRISP-DM

CRISP-DM is a standardized process model according to Chapman and, with its common approaches, is one of the most widespread analysis models in data mining. as the name suggests, the cross-industries standard process can be used in almost any industry and in any area of application.[33] According to Chapman, the cycle of a CRISP data mining project is generally divided into six phases. It is not necessary to go through this cycle in a stringent manner. It is an openly conceived process model. After the completion of a phase, it is possible that the resulting outcome will make it necessary to go back one step or even two steps in the model in order to be able to work optimally.[34]

This figure has been removed by GRIN for copyright reasons.

Figure 5: Phases of CRISP DM reference model[35]

---

[32] cf. Runkler (2015), p.2.

[33] cf. Schacht (2019), p.112.

[34] cf. Chapman et al. (n.d), p.10.

[35] cf. Chapi (2021), p.10

The first phase of the CRISP process model is Business Understanding. It starts the analysis process. Here, the current situation of the company is first assessed in order to know, for example, how much resource is available to the company and also to conclude how much additional is ultimately needed.[36] In the phase of business understanding, it is also important to agree on and define a goal to be achieved through the data mining process. It should be determined what kind of data mining (whether pattern recognition or other classification) is needed and what particular focus criteria (for example, the precision of the analysis) should be worked with. Finally, a firm project plan should be developed.[37] The next phase is called Data Understanding. This is about compiling and searching available data from a variety of sources.[38]This data is filtered according to the previously clarified criteria and goals, analyzed, and checked for project relevance. Through the targeted and detailed processing and sifting of the data set, statistics or similar tools are used, among other things. In the process, possible quality deficiencies in the data also come to light, which then needs to be addressed accordingly. Data preparation aims to prepare the data so that they are useful in the following phases and can be used without hesitation thanks to previous quality checks.[39] Whether the data have to be transformed or simply their format has to be changed (i.e. their data type) is recognized and carried out in this phase. This happens, for example, through normalization or aggregation of the data, for which matrices are usually used.[40] In the application case of economic problems, it is common to use one or more of many modeling techniques in the context of data mining. Sometimes it may be necessary to go back to the data preparation phase in order to adapt the data set to the modeling technique or the model itself. In the Modeling phase, a test model or a kind of prototype is also created in order to test the model and check it for predefined factors. If several models are then used, this is called "model ensembles"[41].If a test model or model ensemble produces a good result for the purpose of testing, the model is assessed according to the objectives defined in the first phase and evaluated in the following phase. Evaluation is the penultimate phase before completion of the CRISP-DM cycle.[42] Before the developed and tested model can actually be used and applied, it is essential to thoroughly test the model again and check for any corrective work that may be necessary. It must be evaluated whether and that the model meets the economic and business objectives and fulfills them qualitatively and quantitatively. In addition, this phase offers the opportunity to examine whether important factors that have not yet been applied also come into play or whether it is necessary to go back in the cycle again to include a criterion and take it into account in the model. It can therefore be said that the evaluation phase serves to assess the individual results and the project in the process. In addition, the next necessary steps for the continuation of the model are to be determined here. The deployment phase roughly describes the transfer of the theoretical model into the practical corporate world.

---

[36] cf. Schacht (2019), p.113.
[37] cf. Jannaschk (2018), p.15.
[38] cf. Schröer, Kruse, and Gómez (2021), p.527.
[39] cf. Jannaschk (2018), p.16.
[40] cf. Schröer, Kruse, and Gómez (2021), p.527.
[41] cf. Schacht (2019), p.115.
[42] cf. Chapman et al. (n.d), p.11.

The results and the knowledge gained from the previous phases are compiled into proper presentations or other documentation options. The implementation or even complete integration of the model into the business requires regular monitoring and control. Because in a flexible environment like the 21st-century world of work, it is important that the model is adaptable in order to survive in its product cycle.[43]

In conclusion we used the CRISP-DM model as a guide for our project. We started with the Business understand, then we went over to understand the Data and preparing it as well as modeling in the final step. This will be further discussed in the following chapter.

---

[43] cf. Schacht (2019), p.116.

4   Technical realization

The following chapter explains the general technical realization of the project. Therefore it will be explained how ML models are created and in the following how the authors proceeded with the technical implementation of the ML models.

4.1   Architecture

To help the understanding of the technical realization the following figure explains the chosen architecture for the realization of the project.

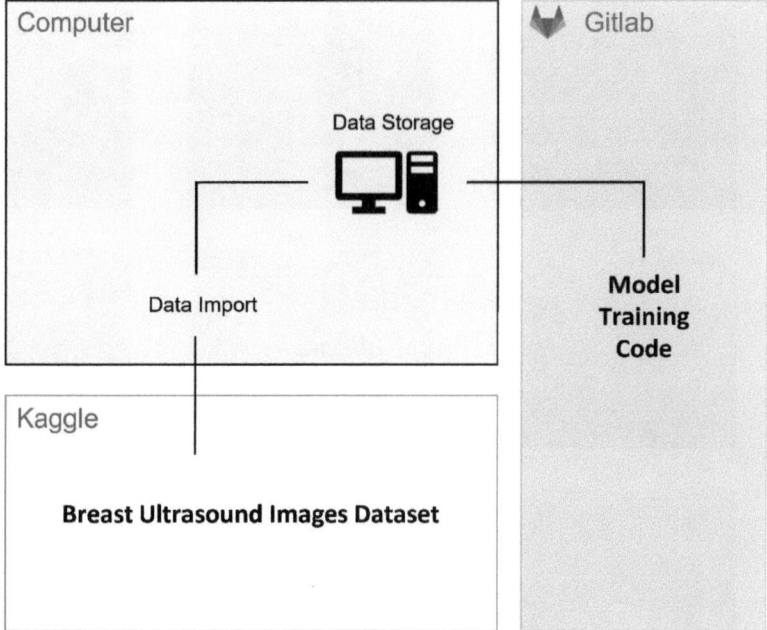

Figure 6: Illustration of the chosen architecture

You can infer from the illustration that the chosen dataset was found on the website Kaggle. This dataset was then later imported to the personal computer, as well as stored. For the model training, the Gitlab Environment was chosen.

4.2   Data understanding

The existing database with which a ML model is trained is one of the biggest success factors for good ML Algorithms. If the data is not of good quality or not correctly classified, ML Algorithms will not be able to achieve success rates. This chapter will describe which dataset is used as a starting point and the weaknesses of the dataset.

The dataset imported was *Breast Ultrasound Images Dataset*, which consists of medical ultrasound scans of breast cancer. Within the dataset, the Breast Ultrasound Pictures are categorized into three different categories: normal, benign, and malignant images. Standing for the severity of cancer. The collected data includes only pictures of women's breasts between the age of 25 and 75 years. The dataset has 780 images with an average size of 500*500 pixels. The following picture shows examples from the dataset.

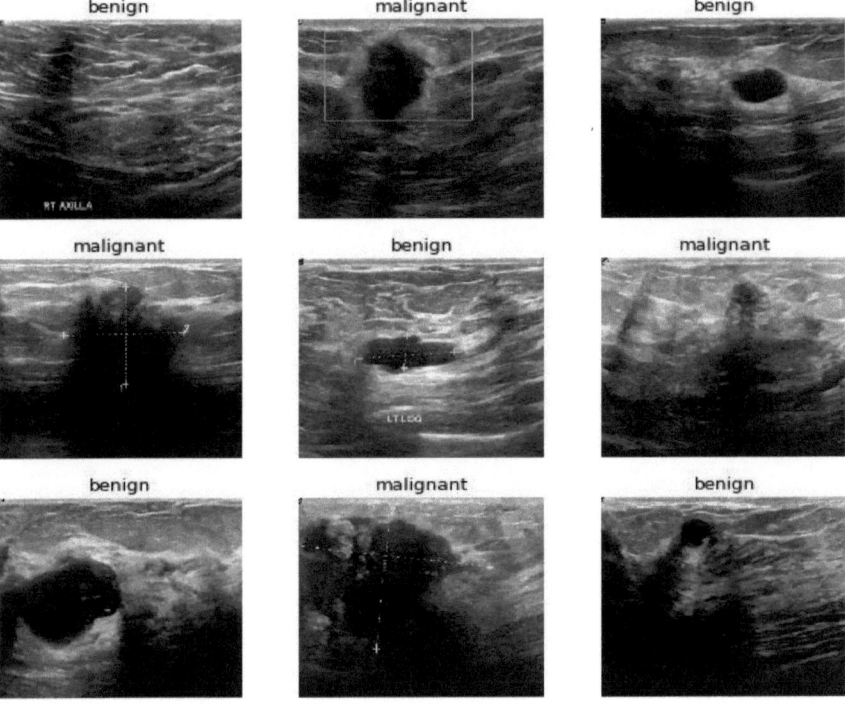

Figure 7: Example Dataset

This chosen dataset has one disadvantage. The 780 images are not distributed equally along with the three categories and are therefore unbalanced. This could negatively influence the training of the models later in the work. To balance the dataset, a function was programmed to minimize this problem. This function will be explained in more detail in the next chapter.

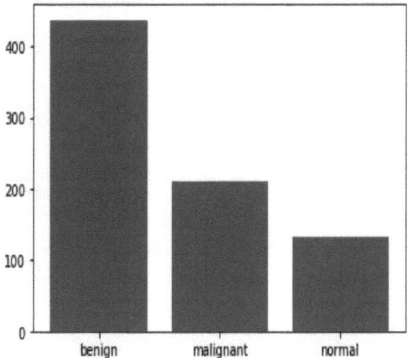

Figure 8: Unbalanced Datatset

4.3   Data preprocessing

To deal with the unbalanced image dataset, the *ImageDataGenerator* function from the Keras library was used. This library allows it to create additional images with transformation parameters based on existing images. The parameters for the creation of the new images were defined in the first step. For this purpose, the variables for rotation, height, width shift as well as zoom effects were defined, which were considered for the generation of the new images.

The production of further images in the context of the development of a ML Algorithm can be done in two different phases. On the one hand, additional images can be created during modeling and training. On the other hand, there is the possibility to implement the image creation before the modeling, i.e. in the course of the data set provision. To achieve higher transparency for the development of a prediction model for lung diseases based on X-ray images, the authors of this project work have chosen the second variant, in which the images are provided before the modeling.

```
1  #initiation of ImageDataGenerator class from Keras
2  datagen = ImageDataGenerator(
3         rotation_range=10,
4         height_shift_range=0.2,
5         width_shift_range=0.2,
6         shear_range=0.2,
7         zoom_range=0.2,
8         horizontal_flip=True,
9         fill_mode='nearest')
```
Listing 1: Initiation of the ImageDataGenerators

In a first step, the *ImageDataGenerator* functionality of Keras was initialized in the source code 1. Here, the *rotation_range* of 10 was chosen, which stands for a random rotation of an image by 10%. Furthermore, a height as well as width shift of 20% was defined with the variables *height_shift_range* and *width_shift_range*. The variable *shear_range* is used with the value 20% to adjust the angle. The value *True* for the variable *horizontal_flip* indicates that a random horizontal rotation is performed. The last variable *fill_mode* is used within the *ImageDataGenerator* functionality to determine the limit value of an input. The value *nearest* is used here as a parameter to determine the threshold based on the closest value.

To use the developed image expansion function, based on the Keras *ImageDataGenerator* library, three input parameters are expected. Here, the input file path where the image classes of the model are located with the variable *in_path*. The output file path with the variable *out_path* specifies the file path where the newly created images of the *ImagaDataGenerator* function will be stored. The last input value, the final file path with the variable *final_path*, is used for combining the input and output image files.

This together was necessary to get the dataset from unbalanced with 780 images to a balanced dataset that now consists of 1310 images. You can see the difference if you compare figure 8 to figure 9

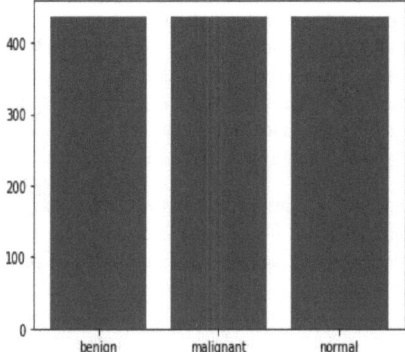

Figure 9: Balanced Datatset

4.4 Functions for creating and evaluating ML models

Since the authors are creating and evaluating multiple models in this work, it was decided to create two classes that can be reused for each model. Changes to the generic model can therefore be made more easily and do not need to be replicated for each model.

4.4.1 ModelMaker Class

The ModelMaker class shall contain all functions and attributes needed for creating and learning a model. First the constructor *ModelEvaluator* is executed in the ___init___ class. Therefore, the respective object of the *ModelMaker* class is instantiated and all required attributes for the initialized object are saved.

```
1  class ModelMaker():
2
3      def __init__(self, image_directory, image_size, batch_size,
           val_split, seed, input_shape, num_classes, model_title,
           model_id, export_dir):
4          # Overarching Input Parameter
5          self.directory = image_directory
6          self.image_size = image_size
7          self.batch_size = batch_size
8          self.val_split = val_split
9          self.seed = seed
10         self.model_input_shape = input_shape
11         self.num_classes = num_classes
12         self.model_title = model_title
13         self.model_id = model_id
14         self.export_dir = export_dir
15
16         # Load the data from Directory
17         self.train_ds, self.val_ds = self.load_images()
18         print('Data loaded')
19
20         # Create Model
21         self.model = self.create_DenseNet_model()
22         self.model.compile(optimizer='adam', loss='
             sparse_categorical_crossentropy', metrics=['accuracy'
             ])
23         print('Model compiled')
```

Listing 2: ___init___ function of the ModelMaker class

In the source code 2 in line five to 14 the parameters are initialized. Thus, first, the image directory is specified, the *image_size* specifies the size to which images are compressed after reading, and the *batch_size* defines the size of the batch in which the ML Model trains.

The *val_split* parameter tells what percentage of the data should be reserved for validation; the seed parameter is used to make the result reproducible. In other words, using this parameter ensures that anyone who re-runs the code with the same parameters and source files will get the same output. The parameter *model_input_shape* must have the same form as the training data. It consists of three parameters, the first two are equal to the *image_size* and the third, tells how many color channels are present in the images. The last three parameters initialize the name and the internally used *Id* of the model and where to store the results of the model.

After that, the *load_image* function splits the images into training and validation data using the Keras function *tf.keras.preprocessing.image_dataset_from_directory*. Then the *create_DenseNet_model* function is called which creates a model.

```
1  def create_DenseNet_model(self):
2          inputs = keras.Input(shape=self.model_input_shape)
3          x = tf.cast(inputs, tf.float32)
4          x = preprocess_input(x) # each Keras Application expects
               a specific kind of input preprocessing. For DenseNet
               , call tf.keras.applications.densenet.
               preprocess_input
5          x = layers.experimental.preprocessing.RandomContrast
               ((0.5, 2.0), seed=self.seed)(x) # change contrast of
               each image randomly to avoid wrong bias
6          core = DenseNet201(include_top=False, weights='imagenet'
               , pooling='avg')
7          core.trainable = False
8          x = core(x)
9          x = layers.Dense(128, activation='relu')(x)
10         outputs = layers.Dense(self.num_classes, activation='
               softmax')(x)
11         return keras.Model(inputs=inputs, outputs=outputs)
```

Listing 3: Function that creates the modell

A pre-trained model from Keras was used. Pre-trained models are Deep Learning models that are provided along with pre-trained weights. These models can be used for prediction, feature extraction, and fine-tuning. From these models, the DenseNet201 model was used. This has high top-5 accuracy and reasonable size of 80 MB.[44] Such pre-trained models are used in medical image classification, among other applications, where there is not enough data publicly available to train a Convolutional Neural Networks (CNN) from the beginning..[45]

In CNN, there is an underlying assumption that every object consists of basic features, such as edges or circles. As mentioned earlier, each CNN extracts these simple features in the first convolutional layers and recognizes more complex structures in the last layers. Therefore, the first convolutional layers for each CNN should be similarly recorded by machine vision.

The authors took advantage of this assumption by using a pre-trained CNN, which is usually pre-trained with large image datasets such as *ImageNet*, and transforming it to fit the new task.[46] The process discards the fully connected layers at the end of the original network, leaving only the convolutional layers (convolutional base). A new feature extractor is then constructed. This outputs the result for the new

---

[44] cf. Keras-Team (2020).
[45] cf. Alzubaidi et al. (2021).
[46] cf. Tan et al. (2018), pp. 270-279.

classification task at the end of the new network. In the source code 3 this takes place in lines nine and ten. Another function in the ModelMaker class is the *model_fit* function. This function is used to train the model. To do this, you only need to specify the number of epochs when you call it. In other words, the number of epochs means how many times the training data set will be gone through and the parameters of the model will be adjusted. After each epoch, the model can be evaluated and it can be determined how the model has improved by the iterative adjustment of the parameters.

4.4.2 ModelEvaluator class

The ModelEvaluator class is supposed to contain all functions needed for evaluating a model. The *evaluate_model* function contains all other functions from the ModelEvaluator class.

```
1  def evaluate_model(self, model_maker_instance, dataset,
       number_of_batches=0):
2          y_true, y_pred = model_maker_instance.get_predictions(
               dataset, number_of_batches)
3
4          fig = plt.figure(figsize=(10, 10), dpi=80)
5          accuracy_plot = self.plot_accuracy(fig,
               model_maker_instance.history.history,
               model_maker_instance.model_title)
6          loss_plot = self.plot_loss(fig, model_maker_instance.
               history.history, model_maker_instance.model_title)
7          cm_plot = self.plot_confusion_matrix(fig, y_true, y_pred
               , dataset.class_names, model_maker_instance.
               model_title)
8          fig.tight_layout()
9          fig.show()
10         fig.savefig(f'{model_maker_instance.export_dir}{
               model_maker_instance.model_id}_Evaluation.png')
11
12         print(f'Accuracy Score: {accuracy_score(y_true, y_pred)}
               ')
13         if len(dataset.class_names) > 2:
14             print(f'Precision: {precision_score(y_true, y_pred,
                   average='micro')}')
15         else:
16             print(f'Precision: {precision_score(y_true, y_pred)}
                   ')
```

Listing 4: Function for rating the modell

Within the function, the first step is that with the help of the ... function (source code row five) the accuracy is graphically shown over several epochs.

In the function, the *accuracy_plot* function in source 4 in line five is first used to plot accuracy graphically over several epochs. In this case, accuracy is a method of measuring the performance of a classification model. This is usually expressed as a percentage. Accuracy is the number of predictions where the predicted value matches the true value. The *plot_loss* function, on the other hand, represents loss graphically. Here, a loss function is also known as a cost function and considers the probabilities or uncertainties of a prediction based on how much the prediction deviates from the true value. This provides a more sophisticated view of the model's performance. Unlike accuracy, a loss is not a percentage, but a sum of the errors made for each sample in training or validation datasets.

In source 4 on line seven, the *plot_confusion_matrix* function is executed. Whereby the confusion matrix is a technique for summarizing the performance of a classification algorithm. Classification accuracy alone can be misleading in many cases, for example, when the classes contain an unequal number of images or when the dataset contains more than two classes. The confusion matrix shows how the classification model decides when it makes predictions. Computing a confusion matrix gives a better idea of what the classification model gets right and what kinds of errors it makes.

4.5   Evaluation of the ML models

The created ML models have then been used in the next step to classification the breast cancer stages. The authors chose to train in ten epochs. After the first epoch, the training accuracy was at 63 %. This value went up to 97% by epoch ten. The following picture shows this result in more depth.

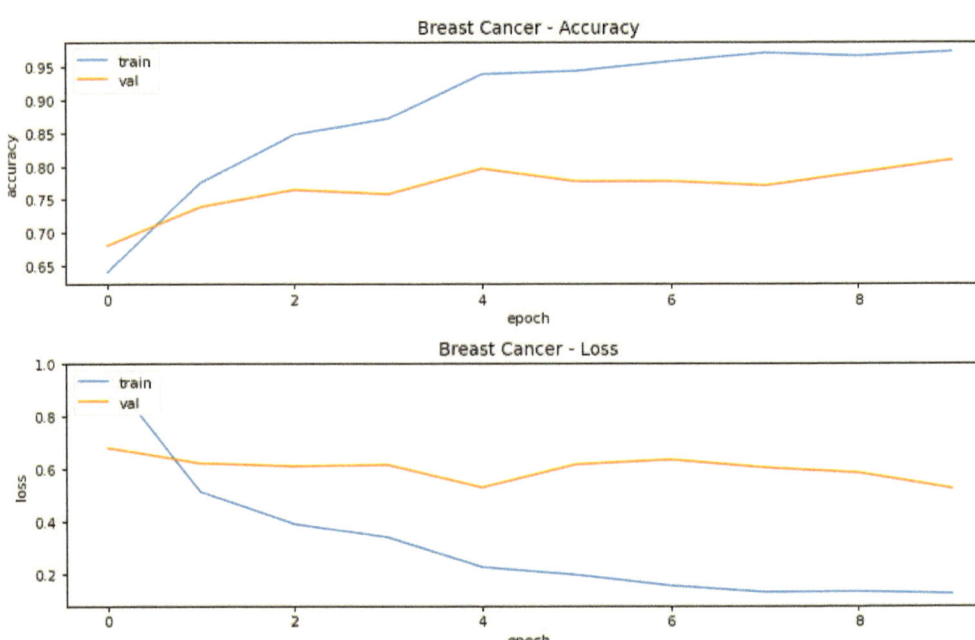

Figure 10: Breast Cancer Accuracy and Loss

The result with 97% training accuracy must be seen with viewed critically. On the one hand, it is a good result but on the other hand, you can see that the value accuracy isn't nearly as high as the training accuracy. To higher the value accuracy more training epochs and more data would be needed. Therefore the ML model is working but needs more time and data to get to a point where the value accuracy is high enough to be reliable.

To look into it in more depth we used the function to create a confusion matrix as explained in the chapter before.

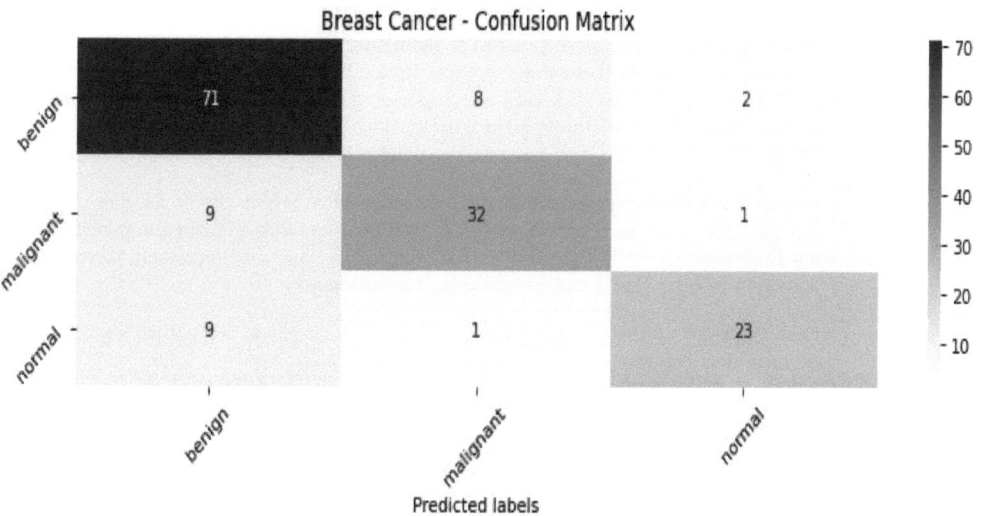

Figure 11: Confusion Matrix

This confusion matrix shows exactly where the model still has its problems. You can see that especially the benign images are categorized often mistaken by the ML model. While the normal images are most of the time being categorized right.

If you would want to reach a high-value accuracy you would have to use a lot more benign and malignant pictures so that the model doesn't mistake them as much.

5   Critical view and Conclusion

To get back to the beginning, the research question we contributed was, whether machine learning (ML) models can be used to categorize breast cancer stages reliably. Our work investigated the possibility of determining the stages of breast cancer with sufficient accuracy.

The results prove that machine learning (ML) models can, in theory, reliably categorize breast cancer.

However, the next step would be to try the model on validated data after showing that the model can work on training data. In addition, to obtain a promising result, it would be necessary to work with more epochs and use more data. With confidence for the future, it will certainly be of help for doctors to use machine learning (ML) models to get more accurate answers, in addition to the classic diagnostic methods.

Machine learning may also be able to detect smaller breast cancer tumors, that are not visible for our eyes, earlier than traditional methods without the benefit of machine learning. Reducing misdiagnoses and at the same time increasing the early detection rate for breast cancer would be desirable goals.

Early detection of breast cancer tumors increases the likelihood of a patient's survival because they can receive treatment sooner.

Thanks to machine learning (ML) models, our results demonstrate a strong impact of hope for better breast cancer treatment.

References

Elflein, John (2021c). *Leading health problems worldwide 2021.* Artikel. Statista. URL: https://www.statista.com/statistics/917148/leading-health-problems-worldwide/ (visited on 01/18/2022).

— (2021d). *Percentage of new cancer cases worldwide by type 2020.* Artikel. Statista. URL: https://www.statista.com/statistics/288551/new-cancer-cases-distribution-worldwide/ (visited on 01/18/2022).

— (2021a). *Cancer - new cases worldwide by type 2020.* Artikel. Statista. URL: https://www.statista.com/statistics/288559/new-cancer-cases-worldwide-by-type/ (visited on 01/18/2022).

— (2021b). *Cancer deaths worldwide by major type 2020.* Artikel. Statista. URL: https://www.statista.com/statistics/288580/number-of-cancer-deaths-worldwide-by-type/ (visited on 01/18/2022).

Chase, Calum (2020). *The Impact of AI on Healthcare.* Artikel. Forbes. URL: https://www.forbes.com/sites/calumchace/2020/10/01/the-impact-of-ai-on-healthcare/?sh=2cb6156a6a07 (visited on 01/18/2022).

Cheng, H.D. et al. (2010). *Automated breast cancer detection and classification using ultrasound images: A survey.* Artikel. ScienceDirect. URL: https://www.sciencedirect.com/science/article/pii/S0031320309002027 (visited on 01/18/2022).

Elmore, Joann G. et al. (2005). "Screening for Breast Cancer". In: *JAMA.*

Mammogram - Green Imaging - Affordable MRIs, CT Scan, Mammogram (n.d.). https://greenimaging.net/mammogram/. (Accessed on 02/27/2022).

Jandali, Zaher and Lucian Jiga (2019). *Wiederherstellungsoperationen nach Brustkrebs: Ratgeber für Patientinnen.* Berlin: Springer.

Staff, Mayo Clinic (2021). *Breast cancer.* Artikel. Mayo Clinic. URL: https://www.mayoclinic.org/diseases-conditions/breast-cancer/diagnosis-treatment/drc-20352475?p=1 (visited on 01/18/2022).

medical, The American Cancer Society and editorial content team (2022). *Mammogram Basics.* Artikel. American Cancer Society. URL: https://www.cancer.org/cancer/breast-cancer/screening-tests-and-early-detection/mammograms/mammogram-basics.html (visited on 01/18/2022).

Imaging, Green (2022). *Mammogram.* Artikel. Green Imaging. URL: https://greenimaging.net/mammogram/ (visited on 01/18/2022).

Lee, Kevin M. Kelly Judy Dean W. Scott Comulada Sung-Jae (2009). "ultrasound". In: *springerlink.*

Paaß, Gerhard and Dirk Hecker (2020). *Künstliche Intelligenz: Was steckt hinter der Technologie der Zukunft?* Wiesbaden: Springer Fachmedien Wiesbaden.

Raschka, Sebastian and Vahid Mirjalili (2021). *Computer Learning mit Python und Keras, TensorFlow 2 und Scikit-learn: Das umfassende Praxis-Handbuch für Data Science, Deep Learning und Predictive Analytics.* n.d.: mitp.

Runkler, Thomas A. (2015). *Data Mining.* Wiesbaden: Springer Fachmedien Wiesbaden.

Schacht Sigrun; Lanquillon, Carsten (2019). *Blockchain und maschinelles Lernen: Wie das maschinelle Lernen und die Distributed-Ledger-Technologie voneinander profitieren.* Berlin, Heidelberg: Springer.

Chapman, Pete et al. (n.d). "Step-by-Step Data Mining Guide". In: *n.d.*

Jannaschk, Kai (2018). *Infrastruktur für ein Data Mining Design Framework.* Wiesbaden: Springer Fachmedien Wiesbaden.

Schröer, Christoph, Felix Kruse, and Jorge Marx Gómez (2021). "A Systematic Literature Review on Applying CRISP-DM Process Model". In: *Procedia Computer Science* 181.

Keras-Team (2020). *Keras Applications.* Dokumentation. URL: https://keras.io/api/applications/ (visited on 01/18/2022).

Alzubaidi, Laith et al. (2021). *MedNet: Pre-trained Convolutional Neural Network Model for the Medical Imaging Tasks.* eprint: 2110.06512.

Tan, Chuanqi et al. (2018). "A Survey on Deep Transfer Learning". In: *ArXiv* abs/1808.01974.